Heart Disease and Chest Radiography

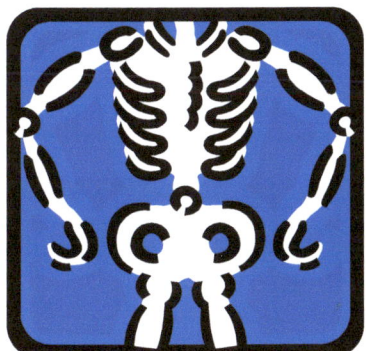

X-Ray

Heart Disease Overview

There are many diseases that may cause your heart not to function properly. Any physician will first ask you for your medical history and what your symptoms are when you come in for the office visit.

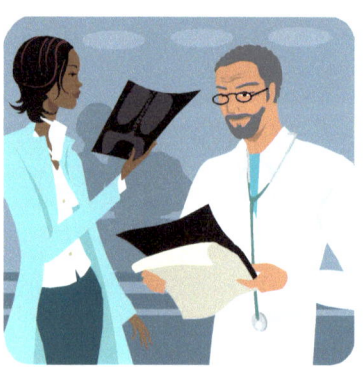

Next, your physician may assess your physical condition. They may want you to have a standard medical examination.

Your physician may also listen for whooshing and swishing sounds to see if you may have a heart murmur. If heart disease is suspected, further testing may be necessary.

Usually, the first test to be performed to detect heart disease is an electrocardiogram or ECG.
The electrocardiogram will quickly reveal the electrical activity in the heart and show any abnormalities within the heart's muscle.
It can show if the heart muscle is weakened or injured by ischemia in some way.
Ischemia is a lack of oxygen-in-rich blood.

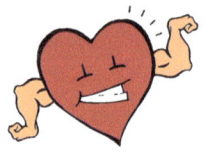

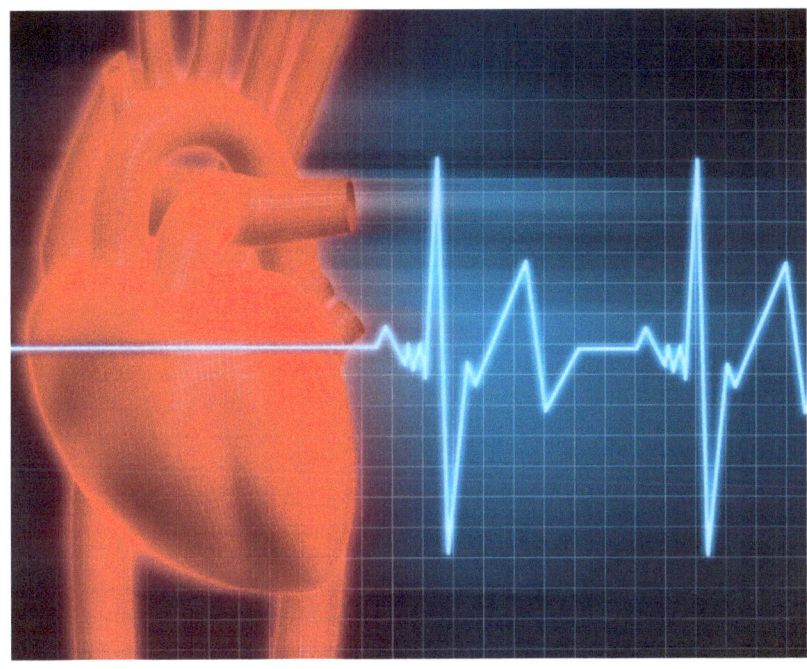

Further techniques and x-rays can be performed to diagnose heart disease.

A variety of other radiography procedures may be performed.

This may be a chest cat scan, an MRI of the chest, Nuclear Medicine or Angiography of the chest to diagnose heart disease.

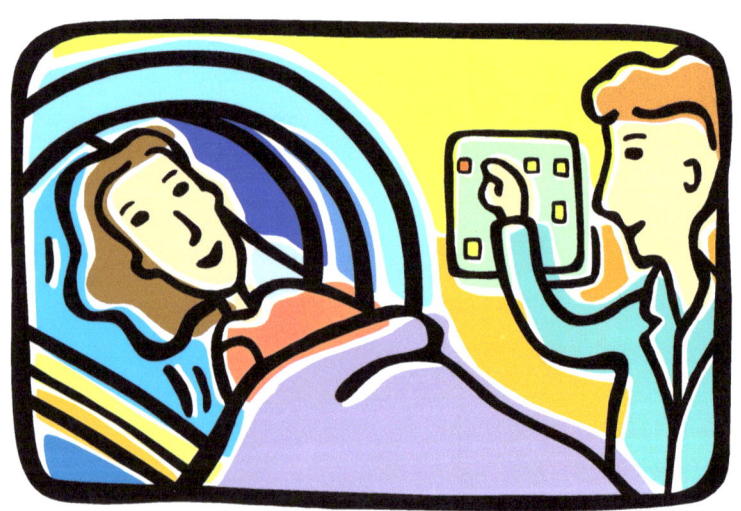

Echocardiograms can also tell if the heart and its valves are actually working properly.

This is an ultrasound evaluation of your heart.

Other testing procedures may be done also.

This can consist of stress testing or other sophisticated testing for arrhythmias.

This is called Electrophysiology or EP testing.

The Treatments for Heart Disease

Once heart disease is diagnosed by your physician, medical care is crucial.

The treatment for heart disease may control the heart disease symptoms for long term, they can stabilize the condition or even provide a cure if it is at all possible.

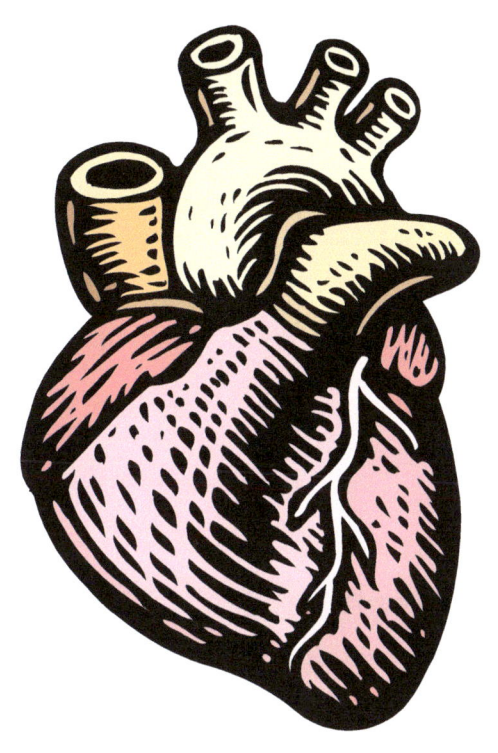

Your Heart and Your Lifestyle

Numerous studies have been done on drinking alcohol and heart disease.

It has been found that drinking may actually may reduce your risk for heart disease.

More than one drink for a woman or two drinks for a man, is not recommended.

If you smoke, you should quit.

You should also exercise as much as possible because it strengthens the heart and its blood vessels and exercising reduces stress also.

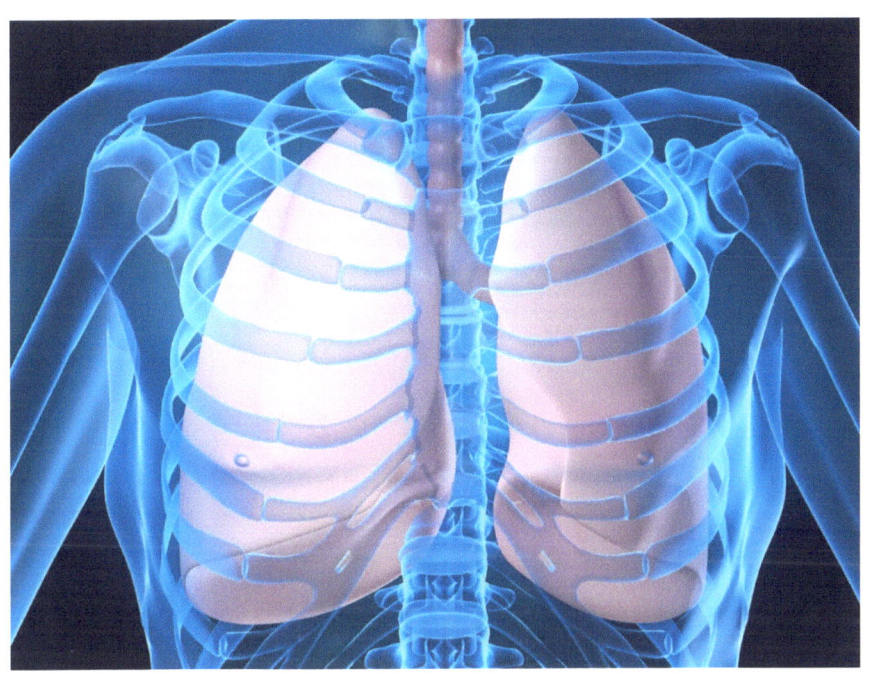

Meditation, Yoga, Progressive Relaxation Techniques and Biofeedback Training have also been linked to reduce heart disease.

A person's emotional responses such as hostility, anger, and aggressiveness have been linked to heart disease as well.

A person may be able to treat or prevent heart disease by simply learning to relax.

A relaxation technique is entirely up to the individual.

Do whatever makes you happy!

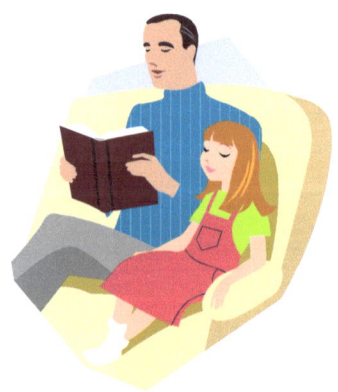

Your Heart and Your Diet and Nutrition Plan

By lowering your fat consumption and sodium intake, you may be able to reduce your risk of heart disease.

You should also try to eat healthy.

Try some fresh fruits and vegetables and some high-fiber grains.

Any small change that you can make in your diet or your lifestyle could make you a lower risk of obtaining heart disease.

This always makes everyone happy.

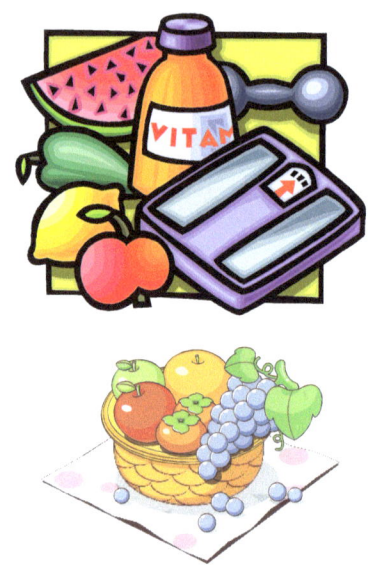

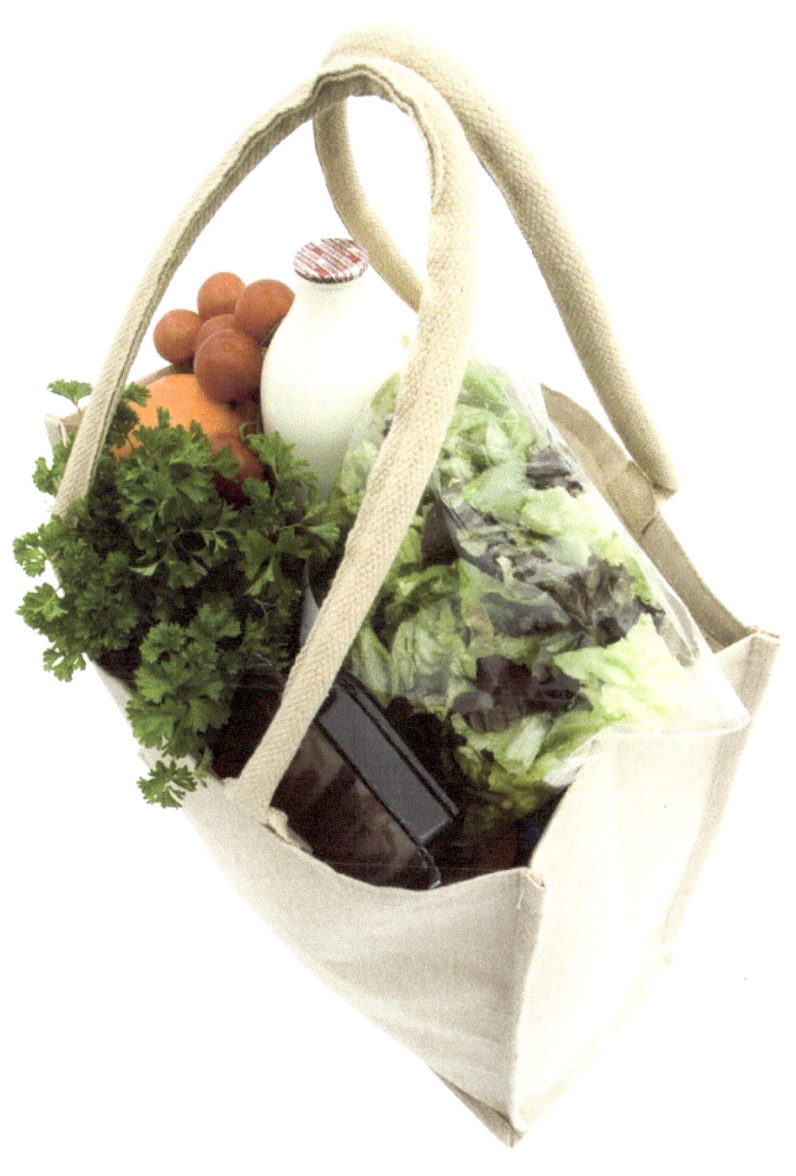

You must understand the Diagnose and the Treatments of Heart Disease

Coronary Artery Disease

Some drug treatments that may help coronary artery disease are beta-blockers, aspirin, and inhibitors.

Surgical treatments could include open heart surgery and balloon angioplasty.

Your physician may also ask you to attempt to lower your cholesterol and/or blood pressure if they are high.

Heart Failure

Treatments for Heart Failure vary because it depends upon what actually caused the Heart Failure.

Some drug treatments could be ACE inhibitors, beta-blockers, water pills or diuretics can be used.

Defibrillators and Pacemakers may be used to remedy deadly arrhythmias and in some cases heart transplants may be used.

Heart Arrhythmia Treatments

Treatments usually depend upon the type of arrhythmia an individual may have.

Beta-blockers to normalize the heart rate, drugs to convert heart rhythm to normal, drugs to prevent clots in the heart(warfarin can be used) and electric shock to cardioversion your heart rhythm back to normal.

Heart Valve Treatments

Certain medications can be used to deal with the heart failure or in some major cases, surgical procedures may also be used to repair or replace a heart valve.

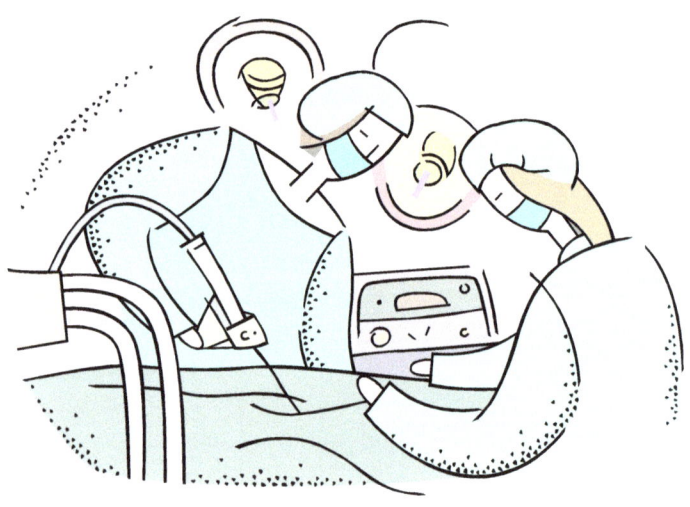

Pericardial Disease Treatments

Pericarditis can be treated with anti-inflammatory drugs such as aspirin or in severe cases corticosteroid treatments.

Sometimes surgical procedures may be necessary to drain fluid from a person's pericardium, especially if this disease turns chronic.

Also, a surgical window may have to be created in the operating room if the disease turns chronic so the fluid can be drained from the pericardium cavity or the surgeon may have to remove the pericardial sac altogether.

This depends on a case by case basis.

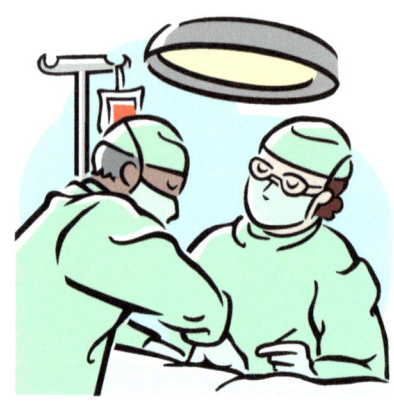

<u>Treatments for Heart Muscle Disease (Cardiomyopathy)</u>

The treatments for Cardiomyopathy generally is by a case by case basis and it depends upon the underlying cause.

Sometimes the treatments that are used for Heart Failure are the same used for Cardiomyopathy.

Surgical procedures are also used but this is by a case by case basis.

Heart transplants could be recommended.

Treatments for Congenital Heart Disease

Minor conditions generally clear up on its own.

Some Congenital Heart Diseases use drug treatments and some have to be treated surgically.

However, in rare cases, no medical treatment can treat a congenital heart disease.

This is on a case by case basis.

Why is a Chest Radiograph used to Diagnose Heart Disease?

A chest radiograph uses small amounts of radiation so that your physician can visualize the chest cavity of your heart, ribs, lungs and greater vessels.

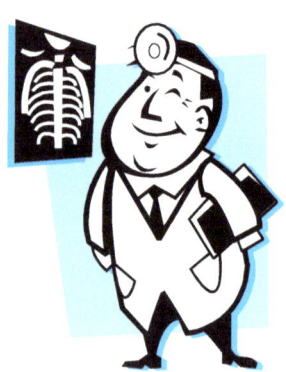

Your physician orders a chest radiography because they want to:

> ➢ Diagnose lung and heart diseases
> ➢ Visualize your heart and greater vessels and bony thorax
> ➢ Evaluate the placement of tubes or devices that may have been placed

How should you prepare for a Chest Radiograph?

There basically is no preparation that is necessary.

You should tell the radiologic technologist if you are pregnant before the examination is started!

What happens during a Chest Radiograph?

➤ Your chest radiograph will be performed by a licensed radiologic technologist

➤ You will have to undress from the waist up and remove all jewelry before the exam

➤ You will be asked to dress in a radiolucent gown

➤ Chest radiographs can be performed at bedside or by the patient standing upright by a chest radiography board in the x-ray department

➤ You will be asked to hold your breath for about 5-10 seconds

➤ If the radiograph is performed correctly and there are no artifacts present, you can then get dressed and leave

➤ You must follow the instructions of your physician as well

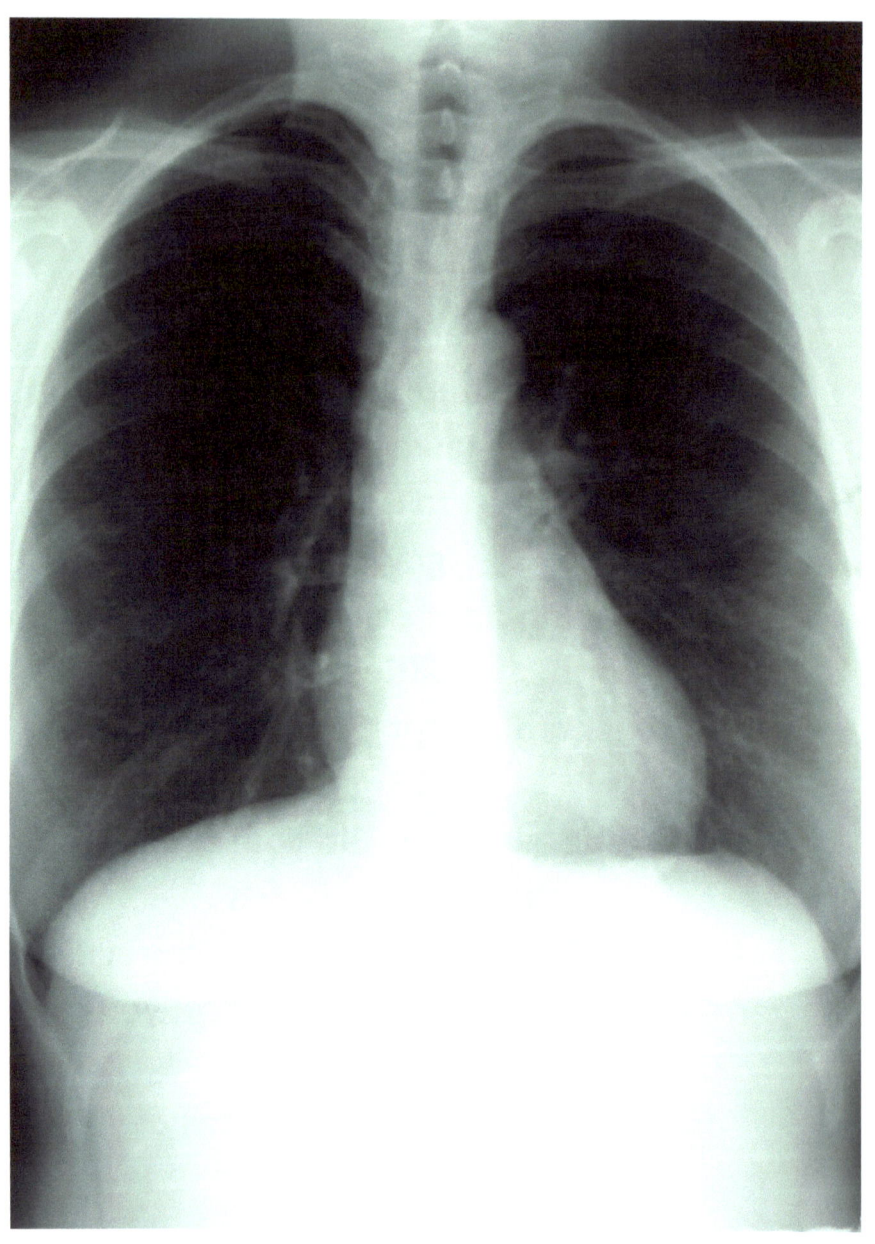

Conclusion

By following these simple self-help guidelines, you can help yourself and your physician properly diagnose and treat your heart disease.

This self-help guide gives you some information on some of the types of Heart Disease, How your physician may diagnose the disease and treatments that may be available to you or someone you love.

Misty Lynn Wesley has a diversified career portfolio in the medical, legal, fashion and insurance industries. She is an avid blogger for Examiner.com and she also writes for CBS Local out of St. Paul, Minnesota and Believe.com. She has again been promoted on Examiner to the AXS unit. She has written several books for Amazon and she and her chosen producers have made several audio books that can be found on Amazon, Barnes and Noble and I tunes. She has also written four books with Publish America. God bless!

.

www.ingramcontent.com/pod-product-compliance
Lightning Source LLC
Chambersburg PA
CBHW041614180526
45159CB00002BC/846